MAINTAIN YOUR ACHIEVED WEIGHT – AND AVOID THE YO-YO EFFECT

AFTER THE HCG METABOLIC CURE

FRANK SCHMIDT

ISBN 978-1-68554-559-8

Contents

Preface

Dear reader,

Thank you for your loyalty. This is my third book that I write on the topic of hCG and I am proud and happy that the first two have received such a positive reception. I am convinced that it will benefit you just as much as the first two did.

I myself have lost a significant amount of weight with the hCG metabolic cure and the hCG bowel cleanse and am already planning the next round in which I want to get rid of further excess weight. For almost one year I have, however, dedicated myself to another project which is keeping the accomplished weight. In fact, I wanted to make sure that all the energy which I have invested in my own hCG diet was not for nothing and that the yo-yo effect does not suddenly occur.

To make it short. My scale still shows the same weight as right after the diet. Sometimes a kilo more, sometimes one less depending on what I ate, how my digestion functions, etc. I consider this success of more importance than the fact that I managed to lose about forty kilograms and to be honest; this aspect of losing weight also got me more worried.

All of us that are overweight know it. You trudge through a diet and are extremely proud when the trousers begin to get loose, and then just after you have ended the diet, the whole fat seems to almost be absorbed by the body. That used to be the case after every diet - and I have probably tried two to three dozen diets in my life.

Only now, after the hCG metabolic cure, my fear did not come true. I, however, have to admit that it was not just because the diet was especially good, but also because I did a lot of things in order to maintain my weight because the big success had motivated me.

Since I assume that it is also your concern to lastingly maintain the progress for which you have worked hard, I want to share my knowledge with you.

Let us do not deceive ourselves, with overweight people, it is the same as with most addicts. An alcoholic will forever stay an alcoholic and even if he did not touch alcohol for years, a single glass can lead to a relapse. It is similar with overweight people. No matter which diet they tried, whether they l lost weight with the help of hypnosis or with the help of surgery, they are always in danger of relapsing.

Although the change of the setpoint in the hCG diet provides some protection, we must be aware that the setpoint of all of us was once far below 10 when we were babies. It can, thus, change; especially, if we constantly get carried away.

For this reason, I have tried a combination of vital substances (as we already know them from the hCG bowel cleanse and the hCG metabolic cure) and some easy diet adaptions and behaviors for my efforts of keeping my new weight and I have been very successful. This can be seen in the way I was able to maintain my weight and also in the way that I nowadays am fitter and happier and that I appear ten years younger to my surroundings.

I wholeheartedly wish you the same success when working with my books.

Yours, Frank Schmidt

P.S.: Since I assume that the majority of the readers of this book have already read my first two books, I will not go into detail with everything and take the knowledge of some basic information for granted. I do not want to bore my readers. Those who read the book without the respective pre-reading can decide for themselves whether they accept certain assertions as given or whether they want to read further details in my other books based on my references.

ONE

YOUR SETPOINT – THE EFFECT OF HCG

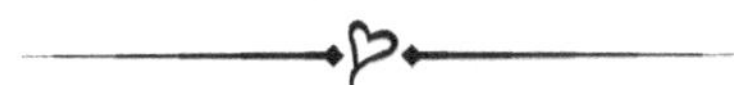

Especially in the book about the hCG metabolic cure, I have written a lot on the subject of hCG. The substance, which was first used in the context of weight reduction by the English physician Albert T.W. Simeons in the middle of the 20th century has an effect on the hypothalamus in the human brain and, thus, changes the information about our weight which is stored in our brain.

Important is the fact that the human body is always seeking the achievement of the »programmed« standard value. If this value (which is also called setpoint) is revised downwards in the context of weight reduction and determined new, the body will hold onto it long as possible. It will make every effort in order to come back to the determined value after a deviation.

Only when it comes to a lasting deviation, the value is adjusted. This corresponds to the procedure which has proven as correctly and effective in the context of growth of humans. If this adaption mechanism did not exist, our adult body would still fight to maintain the weight of us as babies and, thereby, completely counteract a healthy growth.

The substance hCG, which is used in the context of the hCG metabolic cure and the hCG bowel cleanse, has determined the setpoint on the new level, achieved with the help of the diet. Thousands of people have made this experience. Precondition is the consistent intake of hCG for at least 21 days and that a good quality hCG has been used. hCG is now being offered by various producers as homeopathic drops or globules.

Those who, however, overstretch the buffer effect of the setpoint already shortly after the diet due to significant and persistent overeating, will virtually drag it along and, therefore, set an even higher setpoint.

From that perspective, the setpoint can be seen as a significant support with maintaining the new, lower weight. But not as an absolute guarantee. The hCG metabolic cure and the hCG bowel cleanse are also important and successful because they do not only adjust the setpoint but also support us in changing our eating habits.

Exactly in this context, the following topics are important. They are supposed to give you guiding principles on how to adjust and optimize your eating habits without, thereby, living on a permanent diet.

I admit that I got carried away from time to time. This includes eating fast food or feasting from time to time. A healthy body can get through that. It is not about some few exceptions.

TWO

THE PROPER NUTRITION

As part of the hCG metabolic cure, you have ideally made some dietary adjustments. You have significantly reduced your consumption of carbohydrates and also, the intake of fat and calories should be considerably less than what you consumed before the diet.

With regard to the sustainability of the diet, stabilization and testing phase play an especially important role. This is partly about fixing the achieved setpoint and also about finding out how your body reacts to certain products. By implementing these insights, you have already won a number of things.

Most important for the sustainable diet success, is to implement the won insights and also to listen to your body in general. You should now have a much better »rapport« with it and it should be easier for you to feel what it needs, what it gets - or not gets.

My strategy of the lasting optimization of my body is based on three pillars. It is not least about compensating the exploitation that decades of overweight have done to my body. The three pillars are:

1. Optimization of the metabolism
2. Reduction of carbohydrates
3. Usage of high-quality proteins

Optimization of the metabolism

The central concern with a diet, but also afterwards, for people with the tendency towards overweight should be to burn as many calories as possible. In the context of your hCG metabolic cure, you have undoubtedly already made extensive experiences with that topic.

The following foods have a special place in my diet since my weight loss. This is not just about some crash diets, but only about including these foods into daily eating behavior. As in almost every case, it also applies here to find the right balance. Overdoing is, in any case, counterproductive and only does harm.

Lemon

Those who know a bit about diets and especially diets that are currently in trend, will probably be sceptical when you read that lemon should be an important part of the diet. I have in fact, however, not done a Hollywood lemon crash diet. This one is based, as so many related diets (e.g. the pineapple diet etc.), on a targeted malnutrition. That can in the best case bring a short-term loss of a few kilos, but will lead to physical damage and in many cases to an accelerated weight gain once the diet is over if it is done for a longer time.

The lemon has besides many positive vital substances, in fact, two properties that have become more and more important to me over the last months:

- Lemons taste sour, but are metabolized as alkalines and, therefore, act against an overacidification of the body.
- Lemons encourage the metabolism and, thereby, the burning of fats.

Science has long proven that the majority of people are suffering from a constant overacidification. Overacidification slows down the decomposition and utilization of fat and carbohydrates and reduces the metabolic rate.

The excess is associated with the fact that many people mainly drink carbonated water and coffee. But also many more cherished foods increase acid levels:

1. animal proteins, such as meat, sausage, fish and eggs
2. dairy and most dairy products
3. soy products
4. pasta and pastries
5. sweet desserts
6. coffee
7. alcohol
8. nicotine
9. synthetic food additives, such as preservatives, artificial colors, flavor enhancers (glutamate), sweeteners, such as e.g. aspartame, etc.

Additionally, to the mentioned foods also anxiety, worries, anger and negative thoughts lead to an overacidification.

Overacidification, on the other hand, results in diseases and in many cases also in overweight.

Every day, I drank the juice (incl. pulp) of two to three freshly squeezed lemons, diluted with tap water over the course of the day. Of course, I did not sweeten this »lemonade«. What seemed quite sour during the first few days, had become a habit after a good week and had an invigorating and refreshing effect.

Also, the metabolism stimulating effect of lemons is undisputed and has the result that calories are burned faster.

The juice of three lemons can undoubtedly not compensate for all of the other diet sins. In combination with an adjusted, reasonable diet it, however, offers a wonderful addition.

Those who buy lemons of organic quality (which should be self-evident) can optionally pour hot water on the lemon zest and brew it as a tea or grate it and use it as a spice. In both cases, it has a digestive effect.

Cayenne pepper

You previously avoided cayenne pepper. It is too hot for you? I truly understand that. For me, it was quite similar. Although it was not too hot for me, I found that it was too much for most of what I ate.

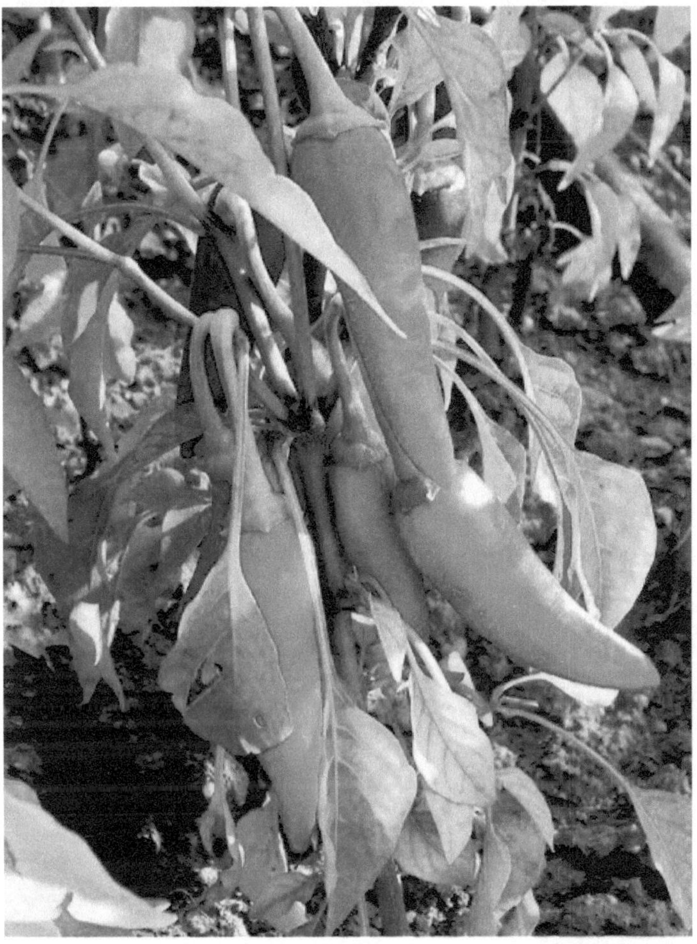

Only an article in the magazine »Fokus« made me use this spice regularly. In the year 2011 the magazines had the title: »Cayenne pepper mobilizes metabolism« and the article began with the teaser:

Those who spice their dishes with cayenne pepper, can, thereby, suppress appetite – this is especially true for those who have used the spice only seldom until now.

In the article, it was among other things illustrated that already half a teaspoon of the spice can help to make foods burn considerably quicker, especially, if the person is not used to it. It was also mentioned that the capsaicin, which is contained in it, has the result that it appeases hunger. It is recommended to not use capsules because the burning sensation on the tongue is part of the desired effect.

Since I came across the online version of the article a few months ago, I started to use cayenne pepper (where it kind of fits) and I can confirm from my own experience that I could detect the positive effect on my feeling of hunger myself and that I have the impression that it is good for me. I, however, only use it in big amounts when it fits. Another advantage has been found because I, thereby, reduced my salt intake which is also helpful to health.

Herbs

Those who flavor with herbs, do in general not only need less salt, but it also provides one's body with valuable additives. Requirement, thereby, is that fresh herbs need to be used which can either be home-grown or purchased as plants in garden centers, but not dried herb mummies. Only fresh herbs provide the whole content of vital substances. Thereby, it is important when preparing that the herbs are tendentially used rather late in order to harm the taste and the ingredients as little as possible during the cooking process.

Many herbs have a very positive effect on digestion and metabolism. That includes:

- Onion and garlic contain not only natural antibiotics but also support a healthy enteric flora which plays an important role with egestion of waste products and toxins.
- Chili, pepper, rosemary, horseradish and ginger have a disinfectant effect, stimulate the blood flow and can directly stimulate metabolism with the food.
- Dill, fennel, lavender, lovage, thyme, marjoram and oregano have strong digestive effects.
- Ramson has an effective curative effect on atherosclerosis, hypertension, and intestinal diseases. It, moreover, stimulates metabolism and has a positive effect on cholesterol levels.

Ginger

Some might know ginger in the form of ginger tea for colds or as a garnish in a sushi restaurant. The famous TV chef Alfons Schubek once said:

»I will exaggerate and say: If you season properly, you cannot ever become sick. But people prefer taking pills, which is more convenient. The poor doctor must then fix everything.«

This quote is from him as well:

»The ginger water keeps metabolism on the go throughout the whole day. For that, wash the ginger, thinly slice it without peeling it – 3 to 5 slices per glass – and then pour water (still or sparkling) on it. The ginger stays in the glass and from time to time the glass needs to be refilled with water. The ginger is not peeled because many valuable ingredients are concentrated close to the skin.«

I have tried it out myself and I can fully agree with him. I like to switch between drinking ginger water and lemon water. On one day I will drink one and on the other day the other. On the one hand, this brings a certain variety and, on the other hand, do both plants contain different further substances, resulting in a better overall care.

Reduction of carbohydrates

One might find completely different information about carbohydrates. Just as many diets can be found, which are either based on a very high supply of carbohydrates or based on low carb (and therefore, on as little carbohydrates as possible). I tend to think of the last one as more comprehensible because it is better justified than the other one and I think of a possibly high supply of carbohydrates as malnutrition.

If we take a look at human history, the supply of carbohydrates was always rather low. Humans lived on berries, mushrooms and fruits as well as hunted game. It was like this for thousands of years. Agriculture, on the other hand, has only existed on this planet for ten thousand years, thus, a fraction of time. Our digestive system and our metabolism are obviously designed for living beings that live on relatively small amounts of carbohydrates.

The fact that the human body needs less energy for the process of burning carbohydrates than for burning fat is a proven. Accordingly, all ingested fats will be »stored for bad days« as long as there is a sufficient amount of carbohydrates. It is exactly this, what stands in the way of maintaining the achieved weight.

For this reason, I almost completely avoid carbohydrates, especially, in the form of baked goods. On the one hand, that is related to the fat reduction, but on the other hand, it is also related to the fact, that these - as already illustrated in hCG bowel cleanse - have a negative effect on bowel cleanse which can in the worst case lead to an autopoisoning.

Especially those who avoid to start consuming carbohydrates after the metabolic cure, do something good to themselves because the negative effects of the »carbohydrate addiction« of the body are then already faced out. Now it only needs some discipline.

Using high-quality proteins

Proteins are a key component of every healthy diet. Besides the pure amount, also, the kind of protein is of great importance. Therefore, it is probably true that several positions claim that the daily consumption of animal proteins is enough in terms of quantity. Regarding the subject of protein deficiency, Wikipedia writes:

Protein has a large number of functions in the human body. Among other things, it is necessary for the formation and the preservation of somatic cells and it helps with the healing of wounds and diseases. According to the recommendations of the Deutsche Gesellschaft für Ernährung, adults should consume about 0,8 grams of protein per one kilogram of body weight with the foods daily. With children and adolescents the demand is increased by 12,5% with 0,9 grams per kilogram of body weight, with pregnant and lactating women the demand is increased by 20 to 30%. For physically active people the demand does, however, not increase. The essential amino acids isoleucine, leucine, lysine, methionine, phenylalanine, threonine, tryptophan and valine must be consumed through food. A mnemotechnic verse for that is: Phenomenal Isolde tryarnishes methmerizing lieutenant Valentin's lysful threams.

A lack can cause the following symptoms:

hair loss (Hair consist to 97 to 100% of the protein - keratin)

In the worst case it leads to the protein deficiency disease kwashiorkor. People (mostly children) that suffer from kwashiorkor can be recognized by their so-called hunger belly, which is caused by an excessive wateriness (edema). Further symptoms are:

- *muscle weakness*
- *growth disturbance*
- *fatty liver*

Persistent protein deficiency leads to marasmus, kwashiorkor or to both and eventually to death.

In industrialized countries protein deficiency only occurs very seldom and also only with diet forms that are extremely low in protein. The average German mixed diet, however, contains more than enough protein with about 100 grams of protein per day. Although, protein powders are often praised as essentially necessary in advertisement, "our usual diet [...] also covers the protein requirement of athletes", says a report of the Department of Food and Rural Affairs Baden-Wuerttemberg.

Various proteins have very different functions in our body. There, in fact, exist a lot of proteins that are not usable by our body or even toxic. There are for example autophosphorescent proteins that result in the »glowing« appearance of some jellyfish. It is an oversimplification to say that the protein requirement of people is covered, especially because the necessary composition of the protein cocktail is very different for different people.

Protein is a key component of our body. Regarding that, Wikipedia writes:

The genes in DNA contain information about the production of ribonucleic acids (RNA). An important group of RNA, called mRNA, in turn contains information on the construction of the proteins, which is necessary for the biological development of an organism and for the metabolism within the cell. Within the protein-coding genes, the sequence of bases specifies the sequence of the amino acids of the respective protein: In the genetic code, three bases stand each for a particular amino acid.

In order to optimize my metabolism, I have, as already mentioned, done quite a few things. But these are only possible if the right high-quality components are available. For this reason, I have very soon started to consume protein shakes once or twice a day in addition to a protein-rich diet.

Since most protein shakes are mainly produced for professional athletes, many of the contain considerable amounts of carbohydrates and further substances that did not fit my goals. I also noticed that some of the offered shakes were not good for me. It might be nice to change a bit around and to drink shakes with exotic flavors, such as pistachio, mojito or the like. Unfortunately, at least the shakes that I have tried, have mainly tasted chemically and the promised flavor variations were at best to guess with a lot of imagination.

Since I already used products from LifePlus during my diet, I eventually remained with the Triple Protein Shake from this producer. This is particularly due to the fact that the triple protein approach, where protein isolates from soy, whey and milk are used, agreed with me best.

For this reason, I consume one scoop of the shake dissolved in 3 dl of cold water once or twice a day (depending on what else I consume).

THREE
YOUR DAILY ROUTINE

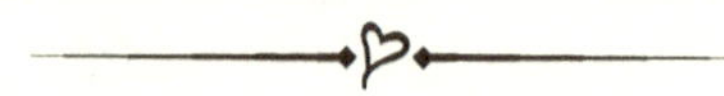

When I look back at my diet, I think that my biggest profit, besides, the weight loss, was that I learned some discipline with the small activities of the day.

Understand me correctly. I am not talking about doing one's work punctually or to arrive in time for an appointment. That was always easy for me. It is about the very little chores and tasks. In the following I want to show you the three most important disciplines because I believe that they are quite challenging for people with a history of overweight.

Conscious eating

Today, I am convinced that people who only eat and drink when they sit at a nicely set table and concentrate on consuming their food, can hardly become overweight. In other words: Those who watch TV, listen to the radio, surf the internet or play while eating are at an enormously high risk of getting overweight. The risk is even higher when any foods are stuffed into one's face while watching television.

I am not talking about the seldom breakfast in bed or a hotdog while watching a football match but about what kind of is »standard«.

There are several reasons for that. The undoubtedly most important with that is that we get distracted by the TV, the radio, etc. and do not perceive what our body tries to tell us so that we eat until the chips bag is empty or the bar of chocolate is eaten. Thereby, the risk of eating too much and consuming the for our body wrong things increases significantly.

We also do not really notice the taste and accordingly feel no »mental saturation«. Eating is a sensual act and if we deprive our body of the experience of tasting and smelling, he will ask for more in order to satisfy his needs.

Equally as important is, however, that the types of foods which we consume »on the side« in most cases differ from what we consume when we »eat a whole meal«. The proportion of vegetables and fruits decreases and the fat and carbohydrate content increases.

One last aspect of eating »on the side« is bolting. If we do not concentrate on our food, there is the risk of chewing it insufficiently and, thus, not mixing it with enough saliva, which can in the further process of digestion lead to problems.

If you manage to eat consciously, you will eat less, healthier and also more slowly. All of this has a positive effect on our body, our health, and our weight.

The aspect of doing sports

Sport has never been my thing and I admit that it is still the same. Nevertheless, I, however, move considerably more. Since I am able to climb stairs without »melting« when I am at the top of them, I use the elevator or the escalator less often.

It is far more important that I more often walk. I am not talking about jogging or marathons, but simply about ditching the car when it comes to shorter distances and also about going on a walk for at least an hour two to three times a week.

Of course, it would not be bad to exercise more - on the contrary: exercising at a healthy rate is probably one of the best recipes for sustainably maintaining weight. On the other hand, have only reduced some weight and not experiences an epiphany.

I could not break habits that I have built over the course of forty years - just like the dislike of exercising - within a few months. What the future will bring? - We will see. Should you be better, stronger and more disciplined than me in this respect - do not feel restrained from trying to exercise.

I, for one, enjoy relaxing in the open air while taking walks and short hikes and to, thereby, make my body more mobile and with the time I might do even more... With that, it is important to me that I achieve a certain pleasure from exercising, which motivates me to go on and gradually become more active.

Breathing

How does one extinguish a fire in the quickest and most effective way? By cutting off its oxygen supply. Fire needs oxygen in order to burn. Children learn this at school very early. This is, in fact, not only the case when it comes to extinguishing a fire or a candle. Very similar processes also take place in our body.

To simplify it, one could say that during the metabolism high-energy raw materials are in the cells converted into energy, lower-energy substances and carbon dioxide with the help of oxygen. The obtained energy is used by the body for carrying out its tasks from breathing to digesting to thinking, walking and procreating.

Our experience shows that fire which has not enough oxygen, burns less and that a fire which is supplied with additional oxygen, (e.g. when a door is opened during an indoor fire) virtually »explodes«.

The burning process in our body also needs oxygen and various clinical studies have shown that the oxygen supply within the cells of many people - especially if they do not exercise enough - is bad. This leads to the result that the cells can only »function« to a certain extent. That, in return, has a negative effect on metabolism which, then, can only function in a reduced way and because of that also reduces the burning of calories. Moreover, it is presumed that an insufficient oxygen supply of the cell could also be a cause for further diseases, through to cancer.

Dan Hild explained an exercise in his book » How to Accelerate Your Metabolism?«, which I have been doing for some time now and which I want to introduce to you:

With regard to boosting the metabolism, there is one exercise which you should do three times a day for about 5 minutes. The three steps of the exercise are:

Inhale for a long time and deeply through your nose into your belly and count to 5.

Now hold the breath and count with from 0 to 15 with the same pace.

Now exhale through your mouth and while doing that count to 8.

You should do this exercise 10-12 times per session. After only a few days, you will already notice that you have more energy.

I do this exercise in the morning and in the evening as well as during the day when I have a few quiet minutes, and I feel splendid. What I particularly noticed is the fact that I also feel fit and productive after lunch, since I do these exercises.

Doing good to your body

For decades, I treated my body like an enemy and harmed it with a poor diet, little exercise, and many negative thoughts. In my imagination, my body was a kind of transporter for my head (and mouth). I never had a real relationship with it and it, therefore, was certainly quite neglected.

This is the same or similar for many people that suffer from overweight. In order to gradually form a (positive) relationship to my body again, I constantly seek for possibilities to do it something good. Whether with a massage, a relaxing bath, sauna or something else.

If it is the same for you, carefully get into contact with your body and try to find out what you can do for it as a treat. Once you have learned to listen to your body again and to trust its signals, the risk of becoming overweight again will sink considerably.

FOUR

OVERWEIGHT – WHAT ARE THE COSTS FOR YOU?

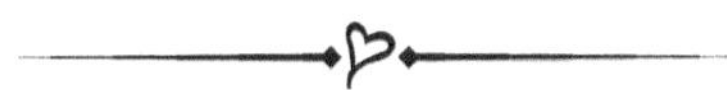

There are many, often ill-founded statistics that show the costs of overweight for our society. One may argue about the exact figures, but that overweight does not only have an effect - not least of financial nature - on those affected, but also on their surroundings and on society, is likely to be undisputed.

Most overweight people do, in fact, care rather little about that. Those who can only hardly or not at all manage to lose weight to benefit their own health and well-being, will also not be motivated to do it because of the costs for society.

I do not want to write about that. I mainly write this chapter because I repeatedly experience that people who lost weight with the hCG metabolic cure, discontinue taking vital substances as fast as possible and go back to their usual routine. The most common argument is then that the high-quality vital substances would cost a lot and that goal was indeed achieved.

This seems a bit to me as if someone would revise the engine of their car with a lot of effort and, subsequently, because of the costs fill it with low-quality engine oil which would ruin the engine completely within a short time.

Have you ever made yourself aware of what your overweight has cost you? Of course, these are different for each person. Some clues for you own calculation could be:

Material costs

- Health costs that are related to diseases and injuries based on your increased body weight.
- It is proven that overweight people are often less likely to be promoted or to make a career. How much salary have you, thereby, let slip?
- Also, the search for a job is harder for overweight people and they are already ranked tendentially lower when a position is allocated - which, of course, lead to financial loss.
- Sports and free time activities are possibilities for building and maintaining a network, which can have positive effects on one's professional success and career.
- Costs for additional food.
- ...

Emotional costs

- Many people that are (considerably) overweight feel isolated and partly limited in their way of life due to

feelings of shame (e.g. going to a public pool).
- Difficulties with finding a partner for life or a chapter in one's life.
- Self-esteem
- …

Further costs

- Reduction of life expectancy and health.
- Additional susceptibility for various diseases
- Pain because of increased attrition of the joints etc.
- Reduced agility and mobility.
- …

These are just a few aspects. Be honest with yourself and make a list for yourself. What has your overweight cost you already and what will be future costs until it might cost you your life in the end?

I made this calculation for myself and have come to the conclusion that the investment in my health and into no going back to my old »fighting weight«, is worth a lot of effort (exercise, conscious life) and cost (healthy diet and organic quality, vital substances, etc.) to me.

Everyone must undoubtedly make this calculation for themselves. I admit that when I weighed 40 kilos more, I would probably calculate differently because I, in most cases successfully, convinced myself that I felt great and that I was happy.

Don't let yourself be convinced by my thoughts, but make your own and after that, decide for yourself. An important step in regard to a sustainable weight reduction

is to take responsibility for yourself and your life. You will
do this when you are ready.

FIVE

Vital Substances

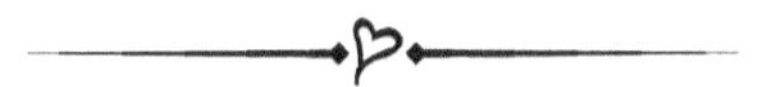

Vital substances are substances that our body needs in order to function properly. This includes vitamins, trace elements, phytochemicals and mineral substances. The food that the majority of people consume, which get more and more distanced from nature, leads for most people to a bad supply of these substances. Independent research institutes have found that the content of vital substances in plants has in many cases decreased to fractions of what it was thirty years ago, partly due to breeding and partly due to »industrial production methods«.

This decline of substance content can partly be supplemented with the help of a conscious diet with original foods (e.g. old varieties) in organic quality. But the fact is, that even in that way some vital substances are realistically seen, not consumed in a sufficient amount. In addition, it can be assumed that the daily intake recommendations in many publications only depict minimum amounts, which long-term shortfall leads to damages to health.

What does an undersupply of vital substances mean? Vital substances are necessary for the functioning of processes (e.g. metabolism), but also as building material (e.g. for the building of new cells). If one knows that a person builds about 300 m. new cells daily, in order to replace old ones, one can imagine how much building material is necessary. Thereby, it is important to understand that this formation can only take place when all necessary components are sufficiently available. The body cannot simply replace an iron molecule with a copper molecule because iron is not available at the moment. Accordingly, a good, broad-based supply of vital substances is important.

Our body »knows« that as well and reports »hunger« when a substance is missing, even if the stomach is already full. This urge of eating continues until the respective vital substance is available again. Especially, when it comes to maintaining weight, one want to possibly avoid these cravings because overeating can also lead to the formation of a habit.

For that reason, it is also after my successful diet especially important to me to consume a sufficient amount of vital substances and to make sure that my body functions optimally. Besides the fact that I do not have craving anymore, this has the great advantage that my body has everything available in order to balance out the overexploitation of my health which happened during the decades of me being overweight, as far as possible. The body has high self-healing powers - but in order for them to become active, they need the respective components.

I am happy to present you, as in my other books, what I have taken as a supplement. Please, do neither see this as a curing promise nor as a recommendation, but only as an experience report. Of course, it can make sense to try what I have done for yourself and to discuss is with experts, such as nutritionists or physicians. Because every person (and, therefore, also their body) is different, also the needs vary and what might be suitable for me, can be too much or too little for you.

Broad-spectrum vital substance preparation

A good supply of vital substances is, as already mentioned, very important to me. Besides the fact that try to consume many fresh, vital substances naturally with foods that I enjoy, I decided to continue taking two pills of the LifePLus TVM Plus as a broad-spectrum vital substance preparation three times a day after the hCG metabolic cure. I, thereby, make sure that my body get a solid basic supply of a variety of vitamins, trace elements, etc.

LifePlus ingredients in ist package information leaflet:
Two pills contains % NRV:

- Vitamin A 750 µg RE 94%
- Vitamin D3 5 µg 100%
- Vitamin E 28 mg α-TE 233%
- Vitamin C 100 mg 125%
- Thiamin HCI 1,0 mg 91%
- Riboflavin 1,2 mg 86%
- Niacin 6,6 mg NE 41%
- Vitamin B6 1,0 mg 71%
- Folic acid 166 µg 83%
- Vitamin B12 4 µg 160%
- Biotin 100 µg 200%
- Pantothenic acid 4,6 mg 77%
- Calcium 200 mg 25%

- Phosphor 123 mg 18%
- Magnesium 133 mg 35%
- Zinc 10 mg 100%
- iodine 50 µg 33%
- Vitamin K 27 µg 36%
- Selenium 42 µg 76%
- Copper 0,3 mg 30%
- Manganese 0,6 mg 30%
- Chromium 60 µg 150%
- Molybdenum 40 µg 80%
- p- minobenzoic acid 2 mg *
- Boron 250 µg *
- Silicon 1 mg *
- Acerola fruit extract 2 mg *
- Alfalfa leave powder 2 mg *
- Blueberry fruit extract 3,4 mg *
- Ascophyllum powder 3,4 mg *
- Parsley leave powder 2 mg *
- Rose hip powder 2 mg *
- Siberian ginseng extract 2 mg *
- Water cress powder 2 mg *
- Alpha-liponic acid 2 mg *
- Choline bitartrat 2 mg *
- Hesperidin 3,4 mg *
- Inositol 10 mg *
- Soya lecithin 6,6 mg *
- Citrus bioflavonoids 17 mg *
- Lycopene 0,4 mg *
- Lutein 0,7 mg *
- Rutin 3,4 mg *
- Soy isoflavone 4 mg *

Additionally to the vital substances, I find the secondary plant substances, such as blueberry fruit extract, ascophyllum powder, etc., especially interesting. These are substances which have until now hardly been chemical recreated and which can mainly only be won from plants. That is one aspect that, to me, distinguishes the product from a variety of cheap, purely chemically produced vitamin preparations.

Summary:

3x2 pills of LifePlus TVM Plus per day (always before meals)

Omega3

Omega 3 has a variety of positive aspects on our health. Those who deal with the topic mega-3 fatty acids find that this wonderful substance is of essential importance to our body. A very well-written article on the substance can be found on Wikipedia.de. It starts with the following remark:

The omega-3 fatty acids are a subgroup with the omega n fatty acids, which are classified as unsaturated bonds. They are essential substances for human nutrition; hence, they are vital and cannot be produced by the body itself. The name stems from the old nomenclature of fatty acids. Before they were identified as such, they were collectively referred to as vitamin F.

This also includes a list of the detected modes of action for the human body. Besides the already generally known effects on cardiovascular system (studies prove an increase in the risk for an infarct by 30% with people that regularly take omega-3 preparations.)

Also mental illnesses, such as schizophrenia, borderline or depression are reduced by omega-3 fatty acids and there exist subgroups that indicate that certain types of cancer are less common for people that consume omega-3.

It, in fact, can be said that there is not »the one« omega-3 fatty acid. There rather exist several substances that are subsumed under the term and which can have very different effects.

I can only rely on my personal experience here and mention that my brain is much more efficient since I started taking two capsules of LifePlus Omegold every morning. When my respective supply ran out and I, therefore, bought and consumed a package of a different producer with another composition, the positive effect did not happen which is why I changed back to LifePlus capsules as soon as possible.

Summary

2 capsules of LifePlus OmeGold every morning.

OPC

While OPC was so to say a synonym for the degeneration of my skin (which by the way has worked very well) especially during my diet and during the first few months after it, it now means a lot more.

As already shown in my previous books, OPC, a substance which among others is contained in grapes and which is the main reason for why many physicians recommend their patients to drink a glass of wine daily, has among others an effect on the collagen. This is what gives the skin its elasticity and the possibility to tighten in the context of a reduction of girth and, thus, to avoid sagging layers of skin which can be observed after many diets.

I, in fact, took the OPC for about six months after the diet mainly for that reason. Afterwards, skin and content matched again.

I, in fact, dealt with the different vital substances once again during the course of the last year. While in the past I focused on what could support me with sustainably losing weight, I was now interested in what I would need in order to ensure a good basic supply for my body.

Frau Dr. Petra Wetzel described in her book »The decision about vital substances« the following positive effects on human health:

- **In general**: Injuries, such as fractures, pulled tendons, muscle injuries, and wounds; exhaustion, fatigue, lassitude
- **Inflammations**: arthritis, gastritis, hepatitis, meningitis, parodontitis, sinusitis, bronchitis, etc.
- **Caries**
- **Eyes:**Cataract, macular degeneration, retinopathy, age-related visual impairment, nyctalopia
- **Locomotor system**: Arthritis, rheumatism, gought, osteoporosis (hardening of the collagen)
- **Gynecological disorders**: Duration and rhythm of the period, premenstrual syndrome
- **Skin and connective tissue (collagen protection)**: Prevention of wrinkling (lifting without laser), burn and sunburn, elasticity of skin, toe and finger nails, dry skin, scar formation, accelerated wound healing, acne, eczema, neurodermatitis, psoriasis, cellulite, stretch marks (pregnancy, cortisone therapy)
- **Cardiovascular system**: Increase in blood fat, prevention and improvement of arteriosclerosis, heart attack, stroke; circulation of the coronary vessels; problems with the veins (spider veins, varicose vein, hemorrhoids, pain, swelling); arterial circulatory disorders (cold, tingling, pain, "Charcot's syndrome ");

edema; open legs; lymphedema

- **Immune system**: allergies, hay fever, asthma, support of the immune functions, susceptibility to infection, strongest antioxidant (protection from damages due to environmental toxins, from cancer, kidney, lung and liver diseases)
- **Nervous system**: Ability to learn and to concentrate, memory function, attention deficit/ hyperactivity disorder, Alzheimer's and Parkinson's disease, senility.

This is the huge »collection« of reasons why is makes sense to continue taking OPC also after the diet in regard to a basic supply for the body. Especially after forty years of stress with overweight for the body, the positive effects on the cardiovascular system were essential for me. The overweight has, in fact, caused a considerable additional burden and the diet was stress for the body as well.

I have certainly not made this effort in order for my heart to suddenly stop working!

For that reason, I also continued taking 3x1 LifePlus Proethanols 100 pills after the diet.

Summary

3x1 pill LifePlus Proanthenols 100 in front of every meal.

Magnesium

For years, I repeatedly suffered from cramps in my legs as well as sleeping difficulties. Only in the context of dealing with my body during the diet, I truly understood that these problems as well as many others that I experiences were related to a lack of magnesium. Regarding that, Wikipedia writes:

Magnesium deficiency often causes, due to the many bodily functions of magnesium, several symptoms at the same time, so that one speaks of a magnesium deficiency syndrome. The complex symptoms include:

Muscle cramps (among others cramp in the calf, cramps in the masticatory muscles)

Muscle twitching (benign fasciculation, e.g. lid twitching)

- *Irritability*
- *Tiredness*
- *Quick fatigue*
- *Inner restlessness*
- *Cold feet*
- *Headache*
- *lassitude/ lack of energy*
- *Noise sensitivity*
- *Rumination*
- *Confusion*
- *Numbness in hands and feet*
- *Increased need of sleep*
- *Heart palpitation*
- *Feeling of faintness*
- *(Lower) back pain*
- *Circulatory disorder*

Moreover, there are studies which at least suggest a correspondence between strokes and magnesium deficiency.

One fact has alarmed me especially; magnesium deficiency is only party detectable by the tests which are usually used by physicians. Regarding that, one can read on Wikipedia.de:

Magnesium is to 99% localized intracellularly. This means that the measured blood levels only inadequately reflects the magnesium pool of the body and that explains why an isolated measurement of the blood level often neither prove nor disprove a lack of magnesium (unless it is a case that immediately requires clinical help and where the body stores are depleted for example due to long-lasting extreme malnutrition or alcoholism).

Since I have started taking 3x2pills of LifePlus CalMAG Plus daily, the cramps have stopped; I sleep better and feel stronger. Because magnesium is important for metabolism, I assume that also have an increased need for magnesium due to the measurements of optimizing my metabolism.

Summary

3x2 pills LifePlus CalMag Plus always before meals.

Aloe vera

Of course, I have known aloe vera earlier. But I only have a real impression of the versatile use and power of this plant since I read the book of Peter Carl Simons with the title »Aloe Vera: Six thousand years of medicinal history can't be wrong. What the pharmaceutical industry doesn't want you to know, was common knowledge during Cleopatra's time«.

After I have largely covered my vital substances needs with the help of the mentioned products as well as my dietary changes, there were two topics which lie at my heart. The first one an additional strengthening of my immune system (since I consume aloe vera, I have neither experiences any illnesses nor colds) and the concern of maintaining the optimization of my enteric flora which I have achieved with the hCG bowel cleanse.

In both cases, the substance of choice was called »acemannan«, a polysaccharide which is found in high concentration in aloe vera. Regarding that, the website Gesundheit.de writes:

The well-protected active ingredients of the plant are located inside the leaves, embedded in a gel which consists of mostly water. The most important active ingredient is the polysaccharide acemannan. It is a long-chain type of sugar, a vital carbohydrate - also for humans. Humans only produce acemannan during puberty and after that, it has to be consumed with food.

Acemannan is stored in the cell membranes and strengthens the whole organism against parasites, such as fungi, bacteria, and viruses. It is immun-strengthening because is activates and stimulates the cells that are responsible for protection. Aloe vera helps increasing the number and the activity of T cells, monocytes, lymphocytes and red blood cells.

There are countless providers of aloe vera products, where some are very good and potent and others contain hardly any active agents. I chose a product from LifePlus here as well, which is called Aloe Vera Caps. These are capsules. I took two capsules aloe vera daily (one in the morning, one in the evening).

Summary

2x1 capsules LifePlus Aloe Vera Caps.

SIX

EPILOGUE AND SOURCES OF SUPPLY

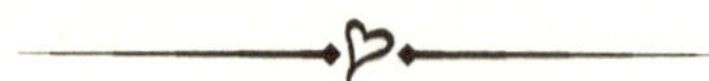

I really hope that this book could answer many questions and that it helps you with sustainably maintaining the achieved weight reduction.

As in my last book, I am glad for feedback and I also tell you about »my« sources for the LifePlus products (I myself am only consumer and not provider), in case you do not yet have an own one.

On request of some readers, I am currently compiling a sheet with sources for supply, prices, etc. If you want it, simply write to:

hcgdarm@gmail.com.

I am always willing to respond as soon as possible. Depending on the number of incoming messages, it can, however, take a few days.

SEVEN

BIBLIOGRAPHY

- Auer, Dr. med. W.: Übersäuerung – die stille Gefahr, 2002, Kneipp-Verlag
- Arndt, U.: Spirulina, Chlorella, AFA-Algen: Lichtvolle Power-Nahrung für Körper und Geist, 2003, H. Nietsch
- Bachmann, Dr. med. R. M.: Natürlich gesund durch Säure-Basen-Gleichgewicht. Mit Ihrem persönlichen 7-Tage-Programm zur sanften Entsäuerung, 2001, Trias, 2. Auflage
- Bankhofer, Prof. H.: Aloe Vera: Die Pflanze für Gesundheit, Vitalität und Wohlbefinden, 2013, Kneipp-Verlag, 6. Auflage
- Barcroft, A.: Aloe Vera: Nature's Silent Healer, 2003, Baam
- Beringer, Alice: Aloe Vera – Die Königin der Heilpflanzen: Natürlich gesund und schön durch den reinen Extrakt der Aloe Vera, 2007, Heyne
- Berner, H.-G.: An vollen Töpfen verhungern, 1997, Medi Verlagsgesellschaft
- Bertram, Dr. K.: Spirulina – Die Wunderalge – Anbau, Vorkommen und Zucht, sensationelle

Studienergebnisse, Krankheiten vorbeugen und bekämpfen, o. J., CreateSpace
- Dahlke, R.: Fasten Sie sich gesund – Das ganzheitliche Fastenprogramm, 2004, Irisana
- Dahlke, R., Ehrenberger, D.: Wege der Reinigung – Entgiften, entschlacken, loslassen, 2002, Heyne, 2. Auflage
- Delbé, J. B.: Gesund werden – gesund bleiben: Aloe-Vera-Leitfaden Gesund bleiben, 2004, M+M Verlag
- Enders, J.: Darm mit Charme, 2014, Ullstein
- Finnegan, John &, Schmid, Rainer: Aloe Vera – das Geschenk der Natur an uns alle, 2014, Ernährung & Gesundheit, 35. Auflage
- Frauwallner, A.: Was tun, wenn der Darm streikt? – Probiotika sinnvoll einsetzen, 2012, Kneipp-Verlag
- Gill, T.: Lieber schlank als sauer – Gesund ins Gleichgewicht mit der Säure-Basen-Diät, 2012, CreateSpace
- Gray, R.: Das Darmheilungsbuch – Gesundheit durch Kolon-Sanierung, 2011, Trias
- Grillparzer, M.: Simple Detox: Das 7-Tage-Entgiftungsprogramm, 2013, Gräfe und Unzer, 5. Auflage
- Jester, F.: Arginin. Der natürliche Kraftstoff für Blut, Kreislauf und Gesundheit, 2010, Verlag Marina Jester
- Jester, F.: Chlorophyll. Das grüne Blut, Verlag Marina Jester, 2014
- Kraske, Dr. med. E.-M.: Säure-Basen-Balance, 2008, Gräfe und Unzer, 5. Auflage
- Liebke, Dr. F.: Doktor Chlorella! Die Alge fürs Leben. Kompendium zur Mikroalge Chlorella, Remerc & Lheiw verlagskontor, 2007
- Loede, P.: Schlank mit Weizengras: Die Gruene-Smoothie-Weizengras-Kur, CreateSpace, 2014

- Lohmann, M.: Der Basen-Doktor. Basische Ernährung: gezielte Hilfe bei den häufigsten Beschwerden, 2013, Trias, 2. vollst. überarb. Auflage
- Meyer, Marianne E.: Sonnenkraft mit dem blaugrünen Lichtträger Spirulina, 2002, Windpferd, 2. Auflage
- Mutter, Dr. J.: Grün essen!: Die Gesundheitsrevolution auf Ihrem Teller, 2013, VAK, 3. Auflage
- Opitz, Ch.: Befreite Ernährung, 2013, H. Nietsch, 5. Auflage
- Oppermann, J.: Aloe Vera – Was die Pflanze wirklich kann, 2004, Lebensbaum
- Peuser, M.: Kapillaren bestimmen unser Schicksal: Aloe – Kaiserin der Heilpflanzen, Quelle für Vitalität und Gesundheit, 2010, St. Hubertus
- Rahn-Huber, U.: Spirulina & Chlorella: Gesund und fit mit Mikroalgen, 2015, Riwei
- Rahn-Huber, Ulla: Natürlich heilen und pflegen mit Aloe Vera, 2015, Riwei
- Schneider, G. W.: Biotop Mensch – Liebe Deine Darmbakterien, 2014, Biotop Mensch, 7. Auflage
- Simons, C. P.: Aloe Vera - 6'000 Jahre Medizingeschichte können sich nicht irren, 2015, BOD
- Simons, C. P.: Chlorophyll – Gesundheit ist grün, 2015, BOD
- Simons, C. P.: Grüner Kaffee – Garantie zum Abnehmen, 2015, BOD
- Simonson, B.: Gerstengrassaft: Verjüngungselixier und naturgesunder Power-Drink. Wildpferd, 15. Auflage, 2012
- Simonson, B.: Die Heilkraft der Afa-Alge – Vitalität für Körper und Geist, 2000, Goldmann
- Skinner, R.: Aloe Vera: The Medicine Plant, 2005, Mill Enterprises

- Skousen, M. B.: Aloe Vera Handbook: The Acient Egyptian Medicine Plant, 2005, Book Publishing Company
- Thust, Th. M., Schlett, Dr. med. S.: Entgiften & entschlacken,
- 2006, Gräfe und Unzer
- Treutwein, N.: Übersäuerung – krank ohne Grund?, 2005, Weltbild
- Ulmer, G. A.: Gesundheitswunder Chlorophyll: Gespeicherte, gesundheitsspendende Sonnen- und Heilkraft, Ulmer, 1997
- Vollmer, J. B.: Gesunder Darm, gesundes Leben, 2010, Knaur
- Wacker, S., Wacker, Dr. med. A.: 300 Fragen zur Säure-Basen-Balance, 2013, Gräfe und Unzer, 2. Auflage
- Wagner, W.: The Chlorophyll Supplement: Alternative Medicine for a Healthy Body, 2013, Health Collection
- Wolfe, D.: Superfoods – die Medizin der Zukunft: Wie wir die machtvollsten Heiler unter den Nahrungsmitteln optimal nutzen, Goldmann, 2015

Disclaimer

Introduction

By using this book, you accept this disclaimer in full.

No advice

The book contains information. The information is not advice, and should not be treated as such.

If you think you may be suffering from any medical condition you should seek immediate medical attention. You should never delay seeking medical advice, disregard medical advice, or discontinue medical treatment because of information in the book.

No representations or warranties

To the maximum extent permitted by applicable law and subject to section below, we exclude all representations, warranties, undertakings and guarantees relating to the book.

Without prejudice to the generality of the foregoing paragraph, we do not represent, warrant, undertake or guarantee:

- that the information in the book is correct, accurate, complete or non-misleading;

- that the use of the guidance in the book will lead to any particular outcome or result.

Limitations and exclusions of liability

The limitations and exclusions of liability set out in this section and elsewhere in this disclaimer: are subject to section 6 below; and govern all liabilities arising under the disclaimer or in relation to the book, including liabilities arising in contract, in tort (including negligence) and for breach of statutory duty.

We will not be liable to you in respect of any losses arising out of any event or events beyond our reasonable control.

We will not be liable to you in respect of any business losses, including without limitation loss of or damage to profits, income, revenue, use, production, anticipated savings, business, contracts, commercial opportunities or goodwill.

We will not be liable to you in respect of any loss or corruption of any data, database or software.

We will not be liable to you in respect of any special, indirect or consequential loss or damage.

Exceptions

Nothing in this disclaimer shall: limit or exclude our liability for death or personal injury resulting from negligence; limit or exclude our liability for fraud or fraudulent misrepresentation; limit any of our liabilities in any way that is not permitted under applicable law; or exclude any of our liabilities that may not be excluded under applicable law.

Severability

If a section of this disclaimer is determined by any court or other competent authority to be unlawful and/ or unenforceable, the other sections of this disclaimer continue in effect.

If any unlawful and/or unenforceable section would be lawful or enforceable if part of it were deleted, that part will be deemed to be deleted, and the rest of the section will continue in effect.

Law and jurisdiction

• 41 •

www.ingramcontent.com/pod-product-compliance
Lightning Source LLC
Chambersburg PA
CBHW051126250726
48655CB00007B/2913

9781685545598